Sugar Detox for Beginners

How to Bust Sugar Cravings, Stop Sugar Addiction, Lose Weight and Increase Energy in 21 Days with the Sugar Detox Diet

Jason Kayne

Table of Contents

Spicy Slow-Braised Beef
Coconut Flour Coated Chicken
Lunch Chili
Slow Cooker Cauliflower Rice and Pork
Seared Lamb Chops
Shrimps with Zucchini Pasta
Pressure Cooker Pulled Pork with Tomatoes
Plum Glazed Pork Chops
Muffin Meatloaf

Dinner

Thai Pork Salad
Saffron Mussels
Whole Roasted Lemon Chicken
Chili Pork Stew
Stuffed Snapper
Beef and Peppers Stir-Fry
Bacon Wrapped Avocado
Aromatic Moroccan Burgers
Liver Meatballs
Dinner Pizza
Crab Curry
Cauliflower Mash
Stuffed Eggplants
Wrapped Chicken Tights
Lamb Meatballs
Tuna Cakes
Chili Tilapia
Shrimps with Chile Paste
Spicy Salmon
Rich Shrimp-Avocado Salad

Dessert

Chocolate Mousse
Pumpkin Ice-Cream
Cacao Bites
Vanilla-Lemon Cups
5-minute Pumpkin Cake
Pumpkin Sweet Custard

Introduction

We live in a sweet world. Every single thing we eat, from breakfast cereals to pizza, pasta, and desserts, contains an enormous amount of sugar. This mega-dose of sweetness disrupts the sugar balance in our bodies. Also, it doesn't help that many of our favorite beverages (even including some "waters") are loaded with a week's worth of sugar. We are trapped in a society where the most accessible high is the "sugar rush". Though it damages our bodies in so many ways, this is perfectly legal (and most of the time, encouraged).

Our unsustainable sugar culture must come to an end. It is the primary cause of the rampant obesity and diabetes that plague our country. We must break our cultural addiction to sugar.

5 Reasons to Stop Your Sugar Addiction Right Away

1. Sugar has produced a large number of addicts – Sugar is addictive. Almost everyone finds themselves craving something sweet each day. This addiction is due to the ready availability of sugar-based products: candy, chewing gum, sugary sodas, etc. Sugar addicts are more prone to tooth decay, diabetes, obesity, and even liver damage.

2. Sugar encourages the consumption of artificially-manufactured foods – Processed foods contain potentially toxic artificial flavorings and colorings. Studies show that many food products contain highly cancerous ingredients, though they are deemed "safe" by food authorities.

3. Sugar overrides the relevance of the whole foods we eat – "Whole food" refers to natural food such as fruits and vegetables. As the sugar-crazed food industry has grown, many people have become dependent on processed foods - instead of sourcing their meals directly from nature.

4. Sugar disrupts the natural balance of our bodies – Our bodies have the ability to regulate, store, and even produce enough sugar. Ideally, our own bodies should be able to tell us when we need sugar, and when we still have enough in our system. Too much sugar in one's diet disrupts these biological processes.

5. Sugar is a gateway to early death – Sugar in our food contains more than just sugar. Sugar often carries with it many harmful chemicals that should not be taken in large doses. Too much sugar (and its attendant chemicals) can cause a catastrophic decline in your health. Many health journals have shown how the human life span was significantly shortened once the sugar industry began promoting the consumption of sugar (and high-fructose corn syrup) in various food products.

You made the right decision by choosing this book. Sugar addiction must be stopped. This book contains valuable information about sugar and its negative effects on your body. In the first few chapters, you will learn how sugar is processed in the body and how it negatively affects your internal organs. You will also learn why sugar is so addictive. In the final chapters of this book, you will discover the benefits of sugar detoxification, the 21-Day Sugar Detox diet, and delicious sugar-free recipes.

It is very important that you prepare yourself properly for this lifestyle change. You may find it hard to cope at first, but you will soon get used to a decreased sugar intake during your 21-Day Sugar Detox. Once you've succeeded at your detox, this book will help you stay away from unhealthy foods and avoid going back to your sugar addiction.

Don't wait – start your 21-Day Sugar Detox today!

Happy reading and good luck!

Chapter 1

Too Sweet Isn't Healthy – The Role of Sugar in Weight Gain

People know "sugar" as a white powder they add to coffee or desserts, scientifically known as sucrose. While sucrose is the most common type of sugar added to food, it is only one of many sugars. Other types of sugar include fructose, lactose, maltose, and even "galactose".

Sugar is actually a type of carb (technically known as a "soluble carbohydrate"). While sugar is most commonly found in plants, animals and humans can create their own sugars from the foods they eat.

Because sugar is a carbohydrate, it adds a significant amount of calories to your daily diet. Not only does too much sugar affect your metabolism, it also affects the overall balance of essential hormones your body needs to function.

What Sugar Does to the Body

This book focuses on limiting sucrose, the common type of sugar we add to our food. Basically, sucrose is a combination of fructose and glucose. When you digest sucrose, it is broken down into these two simple sugars (also referred to as "monosaccharides"), which provide energy to your body.

Life is not possible without sugar. Glucose is essential to body movement; it is your primary source of energy and stamina. Your body breaks sucrose (common sugar) down into glucose, and stores it in your muscles for future use.

There is an ideal level of glucose that should be present in your body. To make sure this level is maintained, your body produces insulin – the primary regulator of glucose levels. When your body has too much available glucose, your insulin level spikes. This promotes movement, excitement, and muscular system activity, to "use up" the surplus glucose. This excess glucose is then pushed into your bloodstream, to be absorbed by any organs which may need it. However, when your insulin level is too high, this means you have so much glucose in your blood that it can't be absorbed by your body. This condition is called insulin-resistance, which causes Type 2 Diabetes.

Unlike sucrose, fructose consumption does not trigger an insulin release. Fructose is processed and metabolized in the liver for energy storage. The liver does this by converting fructose into glucose derivatives and stores it as glycogen. When the need for glucose arises, the liver creates glucose from its glycogen backup. Fructose is very sweet (that's why it's so popular as an artificial sweetener). Most food companies add high fructose corn syrup (HFCS) to their products because it's cheap and can provide a high level of sweetness - even when added in small amounts.

Because fructose can only be processed in the liver, high levels of it can lead to the production of fat. The liver can only store so much glycogen at one point; any excess fructose has nowhere to go. Because the liver's main function is to retain valuable nutrients in the body for future use, it converts fructose to fat for storage. In addition to the dangers of obesity, too much fat in the liver can also cause liver damage.

High fructose levels can also inhibit your body's production of leptin. Leptin is a hormone that promotes the correct usage and storage of energy in the body. When you engage in physical activity, your leptin level rises, sending signals to different parts of your body to release any stored-up energy. Leptin also sends signals to your brain, stimulating the production of hormones responsible for appetite. You will become hungry and eat to replenish the energy you just used up. However, when your body doesn't produce enough leptin due to a high fructose intake, two things can happen. Either you won't eat when your energy stores are low, resulting to hypoglycemia (low blood sugar), or keep after your energy stores are replenished, resulting in hyperglycemia (high blood sugar).

Sugar doesn't directly harm you; it's essential for proper health and body function. However, the improper intake, regulation, and digestion of sugar causes multiple health problems.

4 Reasons Why Sugar is Responsible for Weight Gain and Obesity

While it is widely accepted that eating fat makes you fat, it has been recently discovered that carbs, not fat, have caused the recent dramatic rise in obesity. The following list illustrates why sugar causes so many problems for people trying to weight:

Sugar is more accessible than fat – Sugar is present in almost every food product we eat. Because modern living seems to require fast cooking and food consumption, people often settle for preserved or ready-to-eat foods with very high fructose levels. From instant coffee to microwave-ready pasta to canned beverages, convenience foods have a <u>lot</u> of sugar. Though fat may be present in some of these popular take-out foods, it isn't nearly as commonly available as sugar.

Excess sugar is also stored as fat – In your body's attempt to regulate your blood glucose levels, excess sugar is absorbed and stored as fat for future use. Insulin resistance and low leptin levels can cause a significant change in your body mass index (BMI). In other words, it is very easy to become obese once high sugar levels in your blood disrupt your natural release of insulin, leptin, and other hormones.

Sweet foods are addictive – Sugar intake also triggers the release of "pleasure hormones" such as serotonin, dopamine, and endorphins. As you consume sweet foods, your body will crave more. This leads to a spike in your glucose levels because sweet foods contain more than just fructose; they are also high in other types of carbohydrates that your body will convert into even more glucose.

Too much sugar inhibits your metabolism of fat – Because insulin regulates the amount of glucose in your blood, your pancreas will continue to release it in an attempt to put everything "back to normal". When your body develops an insulin resistance, there will be too much insulin in your blood. This triggers your fat-metabolizing hormones to stop working, because your insulin keeps sending the signal that "there's an energy source available – don't use up our fat stores right now". When this happens, fat accumulates in different parts of your body, leading to weight gain and a host of dangerous diseases.

It's hard to lose weight on a high-sugar diet because sugar tells your body not to consume your stored fat. While physical activity or exercise can slow down your weight gain, a high sugar intake just makes you pack on the pounds. After exercise, your abnormal leptin levels will simply trigger hunger. When you consume more sugar, your body will use this to function, and not use up its fat stores. Your body prioritizes the consumption of glucose because it is more soluble than fat, and highly abundant.

Chapter 2

The Causes of Sugar Addiction

Sugar addiction is not your fault. It is a result of extreme changes in the way that your body produces certain hormones. (Sometimes this can even be caused by bacterial infections.) Cravings can easily get the best of you because sugar addiction isn't a rational choice, it's a biological instinct. Before you can curb your sugar addiction, you need to know how it functions in your body and mind.

High Levels of Pleasure and Happiness Hormones

Three major hormones are responsible for "feeling good": serotonin, endorphins, and dopamine. The main reason you feel good after eating sugary food is because these hormone levels rise. Be careful - these are the same hormones targeted by addictive drugs.

Serotonin – This hormone has many functions, but it is best known as an anti-depressant. It is often prescribed to people with clinical depression. When your serotonin level spikes, it triggers a feeling of extreme happiness. This is why people often eat sweet foods when they are sad.

Endorphins – This hormone relieves physical and emotional pain. It acts like morphine in this regard, and is known to trigger a "numb" feeling. Many people confuse this comfortable absence of pain with true happiness. Chocolates, desserts, and other sweets release a high amount of endorphins, which is why many people consider them the ultimate "comfort foods".

Dopamine – This hormone triggers feelings of pleasure and reward. Aside from being released after eating sweet food, it is also released in large amounts when your body "rewards" itself after positive events like compliments, material gains, achievements, etc. Dopamine is even released even at the <u>thought</u> of a reward. For those who are addicted to sugar, the mere thought of eating their favorite sweets can cause a dopamine release, which more often than not results in their acting on this thought.

Organ Malfunctions Lead to Hormonal Imbalances – Other hormones, such as those responsible for your metabolism, can also cause sugar addiction. When your levels of these hormones are too high or too low, you can have cravings for sugar. _Thyroid Gland_ – The thyroid gland produces hormones that play major roles in metabolism. Hormones like Thyroxine (T4) and Triiodothyronine (T3), for example, are responsible for breaking down carbohydrates and fat. Calcitonin is another important hormone, responsible for regulating the level of calcium in your blood. If your thyroid gland malfunctions, your metabolism may be disrupted, increasing your appetite. Because snack foods are loaded with sugar, you will usually turn to these when

your cravings arise. Once you do, your "pleasure hormones" will kick in and make you want to keep eating sweet foods.

Adrenal Gland – The adrenal gland produces several types of hormones; the two that contribute to sugar addiction are epinephrine (also known as "adrenaline") and cortisol. Epinephrine facilitates your "fight or flight" response, triggering your organs to suppress your metabolism and use more energy. Cortisol, on the other hand, is a stress hormone. It triggers an increase in your blood sugar levels and raises your metabolic rate. When your adrenal gland malfunctions, it may cause low level of epinephrine, resulting to an increase in appetite and high levels of cortisol, creating a high level of metabolism. This causes you to become extremely hungry and irritable.

Pancreas – This organ is responsible for releasing insulin and glucagon. As you may recall, insulin regulates your blood sugar levels. If your pancreas is not working properly, this may lead to an abnormal insulin release. You can feel hungry for sugar, even if you already have high blood sugar. Glucagon, on the other hand, acts as a trigger for the liver to convert its stored glycogen into glucose. If you have too much glucagon because of a pancreatic ailment, your liver may keep on producing sugar. When there is too little glycogen in your liver, other hormones will send signals to your brain that it's time for a sweet snack.

Liver – Your liver processes fructose into sugar derivatives for storage. If your liver is not functioning properly, it can trigger a sugar craving as it tries to replenish the "missing" sugar in your body.

Yeast Infections – Another possible cause of sugar addiction is the presence of yeast in your body. Yeast is a type of bacteria that can flourish in the digestive system - and thrives on carbohydrates. If you constantly crave sweets, this could be a sign of yeast infection (especially if you've taken many antibiotics and antacids over a long period of time). If you have an overly-large yeast population, you will require more sugar, making you crave sweets and carbohydrates.

While the causes of sugar addiction are mostly biological, modern culture also contributes to this insidious disease. At an early age, children are given high-fructose products (ice cream, candies, cakes etc.) as rewards. This affects children's conception of the role of "sweets" in their lives. Children begin to think of sugar as a reward; their bodies and minds become "hooked" on the physical and psychological pleasures of consuming sugar. Remember - the food industry makes huge profits marketing unhealthy food products to children. Be careful - even "unsweetened" processed foods can contain sugar, especially in the form of "high-fructose corn syrup".

After a lifetime of training to consume sugar, you will likely find it difficult to change your lifestyle. However, you can succeed - with the right information and a little willpower. Stay aware of your daily sugar levels, and compare these to the goals you set with your physician. Also, consider using sugar alternatives to soothe your sugar cravings.

Chapter 3

The Benefits of Sugar Detox

Just to be clear, the term "sugar detox" is not really a form of detoxification. It actually means something closer to "sugar cleansing". Detoxification refers to the removal of harmful toxins from the body. Sugar is not a harmful toxin, it's an essential nutrient your body needs for proper function. "Sugar detox" simply means making a significant reduction in your sugar intake. This process involves following a strict diet and avoiding the many foods that contain too much fructose.

8 Ways a Sugar Detox Can Improve Your Health

Decreased Fat Levels – Your body "burns" its fat stores when your sugar levels are low. Fat is an alternative energy source that is only used when your blood glucose levels are low enough for certain body functions. People who have undergone a sugar detox often notice a decrease in their belly fat.

Weight Loss – Because of this significant fat loss, your BMI can return to normal. Not only are your muscles and liver forced to break down fat for energy use, your muscles will also become leaner. This results in firmer, tones arms and legs, which can be further enhanced by regular exercise.

Improved Digestion – Many types of hormones are responsible for your digestion and metabolism. The levels of these hormones becomes imbalanced when you eat too much sugar and you have much insulin in your blood. A sugar detox can bring about a "hormone reset", which can return these hormone levels to their normal states. Once you achieve normal hormone levels, you can notice an improvement in your digestion and overall metabolism rate.

Consistent Energy – When sugar is consumed in large amounts, it provides a surge of energy (a "sugar high" or "sugar rush") because several hormones work hard to immediately consume the excess glucose in your blood. However, after long-term exposure to large doses of sugar, your body will develop a tolerance for it. This "threshold" is the amount of sugar that your body considers "normal". For example, if you eat a teaspoon of sugar every day, your body will think this is normal; thus, your hormones will react according to this "1 teaspoon of sugar" balance. Anything higher than 1 teaspoon per day will make you feel an energy spike. As you increase your sugar intake, this threshold increases, as well. In other words, a "sugar high" will only happen when you exceed this threshold, which can rise to very high levels.

By the time you exceed your sugar tolerance threshold, your hormones will already have been released in very large amounts. When this sugar is used up, the hormones will not return to their previous balance. They will continue to work as if you still had sugar available in your bloodstream. This leads to hunger, sluggishness, and laziness. You will not be able to sustain your energy unless you eat more sugar, which is very unhealthy. This is the main reason why energy drinks have so much sugar. They attempts to give your hormones more fuel to keep your energy high.

By undertaking a period of sugar detoxification, you will lower your hormone threshold to its normal level. Because your hormones do not need to work overtime anymore, you will be able to sustain your personal energy over longer periods of time.

Stress Reduction – Mood swings are sometimes an after-effect of the energy surge caused by heavy sugar intake. As previously discussed, sugar consumption facilitates the release of your "pleasure hormones". When this rush subsides, it can leave you feeling empty or even depressed. Too much sugar also contributes to stress because of fluctuating cortisol levels. A period of sugar detox helps you maintain a healthy level of these hormones, resulting in better moods and a more relaxed disposition.

Healthier Skin – Too much sugar in your body can cause "glycation". This condition occurs when sugar molecules bind to protein molecules. Glycation is a normal body process; however, rapid and huge amounts of it can cause damage at a cellular level. This results in dull, dry, and wrinkled skin (more commonly known as "skin aging"). Undergoing a sugar detox diet can dramatically reverse these effects.

Better Hydration – People with too much glucose in their blood can become easily dehydrated. Sugar disrupts the hormones responsible for water processing in your kidneys. People with diabetes are often thirsty and urinate frequently – a common sign of poor water processing. A period of sugar detoxification can help you solve this problem and get your body's hydration levels back to normal.

Reduced Risk of Disease – A sugar detox can significantly reduce many other health risks. High glucose level in your blood makes you highly susceptible to conditions like diabetes, heart disease, and dementia. People with high blood sugar are also more prone to infection and inflammation.

As you can see, a sugar detox provides multiple benefits. This temporary diet is a crucial step in building a healthy lifestyle for yourself. However, before attempting it, you must know what to expect. If you are a sugar addict who craves for sugar almost every hour of the day, sugar detox can be a painful process. You need the right knowledge and proper preparation to succeed at your 21-Day Sugar Detox.

What to Expect During Sugar Detox

Feelings of deprivation – Expect to feel hungry during the early stages of your sugar detox. Sugar craving tricks your brain into feeling like you haven't eaten enough. Sometimes you will feel like you're depriving yourself of food (even right after eating a full meal). One way to avoid this is feeling is to cut down your sugar intake over a 3-day period before your actual sugar detox begins. To do this, reduce your sweet snacks by a third of your usual portion over three days. This way, when your sugar detox starts, you are accustomed to eating sweet snacks between your meals.

Feelings of impatience – This book is about a 21-day sugar detox – that's 3 weeks of "below-normal" sugar intake. This may feel like a long time, especially when you see other people enjoying a sweet treat.

Frustration at not seeing positive results immediately – Don't be discouraged. The benefits mentioned in this book may not become obvious until the third week.

Withdrawal symptoms, especially during the early stages of this diet – Aside from hunger, you may also experience bloating, dizziness, and headaches. This is because your hormones are trying to figure out the best way to respond to the lower levels of sugar in your body. These symptoms will pass after a couple of days.

You will be tempted – After reading the previous chapters, you now know the many kinds of harm sugar does to your body and mind. Hopefully, this will motivate you to stick to your diet and met your goals. The problem is, most other people don't have this information. This is a sweet world; sugar-loaded products are available everywhere you go. You need to have the courage to avoid being swayed by advertisements for sugary-sweet foods and drinks.

You need to learn to cook and eat raw food – The 21-Day Sugar Detox teaches you to get healthy sugar from natural foods. This means not eating out, calling for delivery, or buying any processed foods. Either eat each fruit or vegetable raw, or cook it yourself at home.

Sugar detox is quite a challenge, and you must stick to it. When things get tough, just remember how badly you want to bust your cravings, lose weight, and have a healthy life. If you can find a "buddy" to join you on your sugar detox journey, you'll dramatically increase your chances of success. Support and encouragement from friends and family can also help you meet your goal and break your sugar addiction!

Chapter 4

The 21 Day Sugar Detox Diet

What is the 21-Day Sugar Detox diet? It is basically a diet program for those who would like to get rid of their sugar and carb cravings. This 3-week strict program will "cleanse" your body of all excess sugar. Your body will have to get what it needs exclusively from whole, unprocessed foods. You will not be taking in any forms of sugar other than those which naturally exist in the fruits and vegetables you eat.

As discussed in the last chapter, this detox period will not be easy. To prepare yourself, "ramp-down" your sugar consumption for a 3-day "reduction period" before you start your actual sugar detox period.

3 Day Sugar Reduction Preparation Period

The goal of this phase is to prepare yourself for your sugar detox and get yourself used to eating only at meal times. It is important for you to reduce the amount of sugar you consume. You must also avoid eating sweet snacks between your meals. To do this effectively, think of every meal that you take and divide it into three. You will have to say "pass" to a third of your normal snack portions – for each of these three days.

Day 1: Only consume 2/3 of your normal amount of snacks (in-between meals), including flavored beverages.

Day 2: Only consume 1/3 of your normal amount of snacks and flavored/sweetened beverages.

Day 3: Cut out all sugary snacks (meals are still okay) and replace your sweet, flavored drinks with pure water.

It is important that by the third day, you are able to "pass" on all snacks. If you consume a snack on the third day, you should start over from Day 1. Don't attempt a sugar detox before your body is ready. Also, drinking a full glass of water after every meal can help you avoid sugar cravings.

Once you have successfully prepared yourself, it's time to start your 21-Day Sugar Detox diet. This diet is strict; you can't eat sugar in any form (other than in fruits and vegetables). However, when it comes to the diet itself, there is no specific food to eat at any particular time. You just need to remember what to eat and what not to eat for 21 days. Here's a couple of lists to help you plan:

What to Eat for 21 Days

Any type of herb
Avocado
Beans
Brown rice

Eggs
Fish
Goji berries
Lemon
Lime
Lentils
Nuts
Organic, free-range chicken or turkey
Organic, grass-fed lamb or beef
Quinoa
Seeds
Tomatoes

Limit the following to ½ cup per serving:

Beets
Carrots
Corn
Yams
Oils you can use:
Coconut Oil
Grape seed Oil
Olive Oil

What to Avoid for 21 Days

Any types of bread or pasta
Rice
Anything that is fried
Cereals
Crackers
Dairy products
Cheese

Creams
Maple syrup
Corn syrup
Agave nectar
Honey
Hydrogenated oils
MSG
Anything made from flour (tortillas, bread, etc.)
Alcohol
Store-bought fruit juices (even if they say "all-natural" or "sugar-free")
Carbonated drinks
Sweetened chocolates

All you need to do during your sugar detox is stick to the foods on the "What to Eat" list and avoid everything on the "What to Avoid" list for 21 days straight. This looks deceptively simple, but it can be tricky, especially when the items in the "What to Eat" list are not on hand. You can increase your chances of success by stocking up on healthy foods (and even throwing away sugary treats) so you aren't tempted to cheat.

Conclusion

Our bodies need sugar to survive. Sugar is a necessary nutrient and you should always eat some sugar – especially in the form of fruits and vegetables. However, you can greatly raise your level of health by reining in your sugar intake. Of course, consult with your physician before undertaking this (or any other) diet.

I would like to thank you for joining me on my mission to help spread awareness about the harmful effects of sugar. Undertaking the 21-Day Sugar Detox is a great way to lose weight and reset your hormones to a healthy level.

Remember - choosing a healthy lifestyle isn't easy. When you feel a craving, remember to focus on the many benefits of a low-sugar lifestyle. Also, keep yourself motivated by celebrating your weight-loss milestones, observing your new, higher energy levels, and sharing your success with others!

Good luck!

Delicious Sugar-Free Recipes

Breakfast

Breakfast Chicken Muffins

Serves: 6 muffins
Time: 50 minutes

Ingredients:

¾ lb. chicken breasts
6 eggs, whole
2 tablespoon scallions, chopped
3 tablespoons hot sauce
3 tablespoons coconut oil, virgin, melted
½ teaspoon garlic powder
½ teaspoon onion powder
Salt and pepper – to taste

Directions:

Preheat oven to 425F and line muffin tin with paper cases.

Place the chicken meat onto baking sheet and season with garlic powder, onion powder, salt and pepper.

Bake for 25 minutes or until cooked through. Remove from the oven and once cool enough to handle, shred the chicken.

Place the shredded chicken in a bowl. Add the hot sauce and coconut oil. In a separate bowl whisk the eggs with some salt and pepper. Stir in the scallion and divide the mixture between paper cups. Place the chicken mix in the middle of eggs and bake for 30 minutes. Place on wire rack to cool for 5 minutes before removing from the tin and serving.

Pumpkin-Cinnamon Pancakes

Serves: 8 pancakes
Time: 15 minutes

Ingredients:

½ cup pumpkin puree, organic
4 eggs, beaten
1 teaspoon cinnamon
1 ½ tablespoons coconut flour
2 tablespoons coconut oil, virgin, melted
1 teaspoon vanilla paste, organic
¼ teaspoon baking soda
pinch nutmeg

Directions:

Whisk the eggs, pumpkin puree and vanilla in a bowl.

Add coconut flour, cinnamon, nutmeg and baking soda. Whisk in the coconut oil.

Heat large non-stick skillet over medium-high heat; place around 2-3 tablespoons of batter per pancake in the skillet. Cook until bubbles appear and carefully flip to the other side.

Cook for 1 minute more and place aside. Keep warm. Continue with remaining batter and serve while still hot.

Breakfast Chia-Banana Custard

Serves: 2
Time: 5 minutes

Ingredients:

1 egg, whole
8 oz. coconut milk
¼ cup water
2 tablespoons chia seeds
1 green tipped banana, sliced
½ teaspoon cinnamon
½ teaspoon vanilla paste

Directions:

Whisk the eggs in a bowl and place aside.

Combine the coconut milk, cinnamon, vanilla paste and water in small sauce pot.

Bring mixture to simmer over medium heat. Simmer the mixture, stirring frequently for 5 minutes.

Remove the coconut milk mixture and slowly pour into the eggs whisking the eggs entire time.

Transfer the egg mixture into sauce pot and set over medium-low heat. Cook for 2-3 minutes stirring often and add in the sliced banana.

Transfer the entire mix into food blender and add the chia seeds. Process until smooth. Serve chilled or at room temperature

Carrot and Pumpkin Muffins

Serves: 12 muffins
Time: 30 minutes

Ingredients:

¼ cup pumpkin puree, organic
6 eggs, beaten
½ cup coconut flour
1 banana, under ripe (green tipped)
4 carrots, shredded finely
1 teaspoon vanilla paste
½ cup coconut oil, virgin, melted
1 pinch salt
1 teaspoon cinnamon

Directions:

Whisk the pumpkin puree, eggs, vanilla paste and coconut oil in a bowl.

In a separate bowl whisk the coconut flour, cinnamon, salt and baking soda.

Fold the coconut mix into egg mix and stir until just combined. Add the mashed banana along with shredded carrots and stir to combine. Place the batter aside for 5 minutes so coconut flour can absorb liquid.

Meanwhile, preheat the oven to 350F and line 12-hole muffin tin with paper cases. Spoon the batter into paper cases up to 2/3 full and pop in the oven. Bake the muffins for 35-40 minutes.

Remove from the oven and place on a wire rack to cool for 5 minutes before removing from the tin. Serve at room temperature.

Crispy Breakfast Waffles

Serves: 6 waffles
Time: 15 minutes

Ingredients:

1 cup almond flour/almond meal
1/3 cup almond milk
½ cup arrowroot starch
1 ½ teaspoons lemon juice
2 teaspoons baking powder
½ cup coconut oil, virgin, melted
1 pinch salt

Directions:

Preheat waffle iron to medium.

In a large bowl combine the almond flour, arrowroot starch, salt and baking powder.

Add the remaining ingredients and stir to combine.

Grease the waffle iron with some oil and spread 1/3 batter over the iron. Close the iron and cook for 2-3 minutes.

Repeat with remaining batter and serve with fresh fruits.

Detox Porridge

Serves: 2
Time: 15 minutes

Ingredients:

½ cup coconut flour
1 teaspoon cinnamon
2 tablespoons coconut oil, virgin, melted
2 cups water
2 teaspoons stevia
1 pinch nutmeg
1 cup almond milk
4 tablespoons golden flax, ground

Directions:

Combine all ingredients in sauce pan.

Bring to gentle simmer over medium heat. Simmer, stirring for 5 minutes.

Serve while still hot.

Apple Cinnamon Muffins

Serves: 12 muffins
Time: 30minutes

Ingredients:

¼ cup coconut flour
¼ cup almond flour
2 teaspoons cinnamon
¼ teaspoon baking soda
1 teaspoon cardamom
2 green apples, peeled, cored, diced small
4 eggs
2 teaspoons vanilla paste
½ cup coconut milk
1 tablespoon coconut oil, virgin, melted
1 pinch salt

Directions:

Preheat oven to 370F and line 12-hole muffin tin with paper cases.

In a bowl combine the coconut flour, almond flour, cinnamon, cardamom, baking soda and salt.

In separate bowl whisk the milk with water and vanilla paste. Fold the liquid ingredients into dry ones and add the oil. Stir to combine.

Finally add the chopped apple and stir to blend.

Spoon the batter into paper cups and bake in preheated oven for 20 minutes or until inserted toothpick comes out clean.

Place the muffin tin onto wire rack to cool for 5 minutes before removing the muffins from the tin. Serve after.

Cinnamon-Banana Smoothie

Serves: 1
Time: 5 minutes

Ingredients:

4 egg yolks, fresh
½ cup coconut milk
¼ cup ice
½ teaspoon cinnamon
1 pinch cardamom, ground
1 banana, unripe (green tipped)
1 tablespoon chia seeds

Directions:

In a blender, combine all ingredients.

Process until smooth.

Serve in tall glass immediately.

Cacao Pancakes

Serves: 6 mini pancakes
Time: 10 minutes

Ingredients:

1 tablespoon cacao, raw
2 bananas, unripe (green tipped)
1 egg
1 tablespoon coconut milk

Directions:

Mash the bananas and combine with egg.

Combine the milk with cacao powder to form a past.
Stir the cacao paste into banana mix and stir until
blended thoroughly.

Heat some coconut oil in large skillet. Scoop ¼ cup
batter and place into skillet. Cook the pancake until
bubbles appear. Flip carefully to the other side and
cook for 1 minute more.

Serve after.

Breakfast Patties

Serves: 8 patties
Time: 20 minutes

Ingredients:

1 lb. pork, ground
½ teaspoon sage
½ teaspoon thyme
2 tablespoons coconut oil, virgin, melted
1 teaspoon garlic, minced
½ teaspoon cumin, ground
½ teaspoon black pepper
½ teaspoon red chili flakes
1 teaspoon paprika, smoked

Directions:

In a bowl, combine pork with sage, thyme, salt, pepper, cumin, chili, pepper flakes and garlic.

Heat half of coconut oil in large skillet.

Form 8 patties from the meat mixture. Place four patties in skillet and cook for 3-4 minutes per side.

Remove and place on paper towel lined plate. Repeat the procedure with remaining oil and meat patties.

Serve immediately.

Lunch

Beef and Cabbage Soup

Serves: 4
Time: 70 minutes

Ingredients:

1 lb. beef, stew type
0.5 pcs head cabbage, sliced
3 quarts chicken stock
2 teaspoon parsley. Fresh, chopped
1 sprig thyme, fresh
4 carrots, grated
1 pcs onion, chopped
1 bay leaf
3 tablespoons coconut oil, melted
2 clove garlic, chopped
2 celery stalks, chopped
¼ teaspoon salt
1/8 teaspoon black pepper

Directions:

Heat oil in sauce pot over medium-high heat. Add
onions and cook for 3 minutes. Add carrots and celery
and cook for 3 minutes more. Season with salt and
pepper.

Add beef and cook until browned. Add the stock along
with thyme, bay leaf, parsley and cook for 30 minutes.

Add the cabbage and cook all for 30 minutes more or until meat is tender. Season additionally with salt and pepper and serve while still hot.

Turkey Burgers

Serves: 6 burgers
Time: 20 minutes

Ingredients:

1 lb. ground turkey, lean
2 tablespoons coconut oil, melted
½ cup almond butter
1 egg white
½ cup carrots, shredded
½ teaspoon curry paste, mild
½ teaspoon garam masala
½ teaspoon salt
1pcs onion, chopped finely

Directions:

Place the turkey in a bowl. Add the almond butter, egg white, curry paste and garam masala.

Heat ½ tablespoon coconut oil in small sauce pan; add onions and carrots and cook until tender. Place aside to cool and once cooled enough to handle, combine with the turkey.

Form six patties from the turkey.

Heat remaining coconut oil and cook the burgers for 4 minutes per side. Serve with fresh vegetable cuts.

Fish Sticks

Serves: 4
Time: 30 minutes

Ingredients:

4 oz. tilapia fillets
2 tablespoons coconut oil, melted
½ cup coconut flour
1 cup almond flour
1 teaspoon basil, dried, crushed
½ teaspoon oregano, dried, crushed
½ teaspoon salt
2 eggs
2 teaspoons water

Directions:

Combine the coconut flour, almond flour, basil, salt and oregano in wide plate. Whisk the eggs with water in a bowl.

Cut the tilapia fillets in a 1 ½-inch wide sticks. Dip the fish sticks into egg mixture and dredge through the flour mix.

Heat the oven to 450F and line baking sheet with parchment paper. Arrange coated fish sticks onto baking sheet and brush each stick with melted coconut oil. Bake the sticks for 15-20 minutes and serve after.

Chicken Stuffed Peppers

Serves: 4 peppers
Time: 30 minutes

Ingredients:

4 red bell peppers
2 chicken breast fillets, chopped
½ cup chicken broth
¼ cup onion, finely minced
2 tablespoons jalapenos, minced
1 teaspoon salt
1 teaspoon chili powder
1 cup tomatoes, diced
½ teaspoon garlic powder
½ teaspoon cumin, ground
¼ teaspoon oregano
2 cups salsa verde

Directions:

Cut the pepper tops and pull out the inside membrane and seeds.

Place the chicken in a sauce pot and add chicken broth, onion, jalapenos, salt, chili powder, tomatoes, garlic powder, cumin and oregano.

Cook over medium heat until chicken is tender and the broth has evaporated.

Stuff the bell peppers with prepared chicken mix and place into baking dish. Top the peppers with salsa verde and bake in preheated oven at 350F for 20 minutes.

Serve after, while still hot.

Spicy Chicken Drumsticks

Serves: 4
Time: 25 minutes

Ingredients:

¾ lb. chicken drumsticks
1 teaspoon curry spice
2 tablespoons coconut oil, melted, virgin
1 teaspoon cinnamon
½ teaspoon garlic, minced
½ teaspoon ground ginger
1sprig thyme, chopped

Directions:

Wash and pat-dry the drumsticks.

Place the drumsticks in a plastic bag and add the curry spice, cinnamon, ginger and garlic. Close the bag and shake well.

Heat the coconut oil in skillet over medium-high heat; add the thyme and cook until fragrant. Add the chicken, skin side and cook for 5 minutes. Flip the drumstick and cook for 3 minutes more. Reduce heat to low and return the drumsticks on the skin side. Cover and cook for 10-12 minutes more.

Serve after.

Turkey Poppers with Zucchini

Serves: 4
Time: 25 minutes

Ingredients:

1 lb. turkey, ground
4 tablespoons cilantro, fresh, minced
1 teaspoon salt
½ teaspoon white pepper, ground
2 cups grated zucchinis, with skin
2 scallions, minced
2 clove garlic, minced
1 teaspoon cumin, ground
½ teaspoon red pepper flakes
Some coconut oil – to drizzle

Directions:

Combine all the ingredients in a bowl; turkey with cilantro, scallions, salt, pepper, zucchinis, garlic, cumin and red pepper flakes.

Preheat the oven to 400F and line baking sheet with parchment paper.

Scoop meatballs onto baking sheet and drizzle with coconut oil. Bake in preheated oven for 20 minutes. Serve with fresh guacamole.

Spicy Slow-Braised Beef

Serves: 4
Time: 3 hours 10 minutes

Ingredients:

2 lb. beef stew meat, cut into ½-inch cubes
3 garlic cloves, minced
1 tablespoon chili powder
1 tablespoon coconut oil, melted
½ cup cilantro, minced
1 teaspoon salt
1 onion, sliced thinly
1 tablespoon tomato paste, organic
1 cup salsa
½ cup beef broth

Directions:

Preheat oven to 300F.

In a bowl combine the beef with chili powder and salt.

Heat coconut oil in large skillet; add onions and cook for 3-4 minutes. Add tomato paste and cook for 30 seconds.

Add garlic and cook for 30 seconds more. Finally add seasoned beef and salsa. Stir well.

Add stock and stir again. Cover the pot and transfer in the oven. Cook for 3 hours or until meat is tender.

Adjust seasonings before serving.

Coconut Flour Coated Chicken

Serves: 4
Time: 15 minutes

Ingredients:

1 pair chicken breast
2 tablespoons red pepper flakes
2 cups coconut flakes, unsweetened
½ cup coconut flour
2 egg whites
Salt and pepper – to taste
Coconut oil – to fry

Directions:

Wash and pat-dry the chicken. Cut into 1-inch wide strips. Season with salt and pepper.

In a shallow dish combine the coconut flour, red pepper flakes and one pinch pepper.

Place the coconut flakes in separate dish and whisk the egg whites in third dish.

Dredge the chicken strips through the coconut flour mix, dip in the egg whites and place in a dish with coconut flakes. Coat well with coconut flakes and place into skillet with 1-inch heated coconut oil.

Cook the chicken until golden-brown and place in a paper towel lined plate. Serve with fresh salsa verde or guacamole.

Lunch Chili

Serves: 4
Time: 70 minutes

Ingredients:

2lb. beef, cut into pieces
4 cups tomatoes, diced
¼ cup coconut oil, melted
4 garlic cloves, chopped finely
1 pcs onion, chopped
1 cup water
1 tablespoon smoked paprika
1 tablespoon oregano, dried
2 teaspoons salt
2 teaspoons cumin, ground
1pcs jalapeno, chopped

1pcs bell pepper, chopped

Directions:

Heat oil in Dutch oven. Add onion with pepper and cook for 5 minutes.

Add the garlic along with cumin and jalapeno and cook for 1 minute.

Add the beef along with remaining ingredients and simmer for 1 hour over medium heat or until the beef is tender.

Serve while still hot.

Slow Cooker Cauliflower Rice and Pork

Serves: 4
Time: 8 hours

Ingredients:

1 lb. pork shoulder
1 head cauliflower, roughly chopped
1 teaspoon cumin, ground
1 teaspoon salt
4 garlic cloves, chopped
½ teaspoon black pepper, crushed
1 teaspoon chili powder
1 cup chicken stock, low-sodium

Directions:

Place the cauliflower in food processor and pulse few times until you have rice structure.

Place the cauliflower rice in slow cooker and add chicken stock. Season with cumin and chili.

Make the cuts in pork shoulder and place the garlic in the cuts. Season with salt and pepper.

Top the cauliflower with pork meat and close with lid.

Cook on low for 8 hours. Pull the pork using fork and serve with prepared cauliflower rice.

Seared Lamb Chops

Serves: 4
Time: 10 minutes

Ingredients:

8 lamb chops
1 tablespoon coconut oil
½ tablespoon salt
1 tablespoon thyme, dried
Black pepper – to taste

Directions:

Place the salt and thyme in mini flood blender or mortar. Pulse until combined or grind in mortar until combined.

Melt the coconut oil in large skillet. Preheat oven to 400F.

Season the lamb chops with black pepper and salt-thyme mixture.

Once the oil is hot, sear the lamb chops for 2 minutes per side.

Pop in the oven for 2 minutes more and serve after.

Shrimps with Zucchini Pasta

Serves: 4
Time: 15 min

Ingredients:

16 oz. shrimps, deveined
4 pcs zucchinis, spiralized (or cut into thin strips)
4 garlic cloves, minced
4 tablespoons olive oil
2 pcs lemon, juiced and zested
2 tablespoons almond butter
Salt and pepper – to taste

Directions:

Preheat oven to 400F.

Combine the shrimps, garlic, olive oil, lemon juice, lemon zest and almond butter in baking dish.

Season with salt and pepper and cook for 8-10 minutes or until shrimps are no longer pink, turning once.

Add zucchini pasta in the last minutes of cooking or serve the shrimps with uncooked zucchini pasta.

Pressure Cooker Pulled Pork with Tomatoes

Serves: 4
Time: 80 minutes

Ingredients:

1 lb. pork shoulder roast
1 pcs yellow onion, chopped
8 oz. tomato sauce
2 tablespoons lime juice
1 jalapeno pepper, chopped
1 tablespoon avocado oil
2 garlic cloves, chopped
Salt and pepper – to taste

Directions:

Heat the avocado oil in large skillet over medium-high heat.

Add the onion and cook for 5 minutes; add garlic and cook for 1 minute. Remove the onions from the skillet and add pork meat. Sear the meat on all sides and transfer in pressure cooker.

Add the tomato sauce, jalapeno and lime juice. Close the lid and cook the pork on low pressure for 60-65 minutes. Release the pressure according to manufacturer's instructions. Remove the pork and pull using forks. Serve and top with cooking juices.

Plum Glazed Pork Chops

Serves: 4
Time: 12 minutes

Ingredients:

8 pork loin chops, boneless
1 ½ tablespoons garlic powder
1 ½ tablespoons onion powder
4 tablespoons chipotle powder
1 tablespoon coconut oil, melted
¼ cup plums, pureed
1 tablespoon sage, dried, crushed
Salt and fresh ground pepper

Directions:

Combine the plum puree, sage and chipotle in a small bowl to make a paste.

Season the pork with salt, pepper, garlic and onion powder.

Heat the remaining oil in large skillet over medium-high heat.

Place the pork chops and brush with prepared paste. Sear for 2 minutes and turn to the other side. Brush the other side as well and sear the chops for 2 minutes on this side.

Lower the heat, cover the chops and cook for 5-6 minutes more.

Brush the chops with remaining paste and remove from the heat.

Allow to rest for 5 minutes before serving.

Muffin Meatloaf

Serves: 6 meatloaf muffins
Time: 30 minutes

Ingredients:

1 lb. beef, ground
1 egg
1 egg white
1 tablespoon mustard seeds, ground
1 cup tomatoes, pureed
1 tablespoon apple cider vinegar
1 pcs zucchini, shredded
1 pcs onion, chopped finely
½ teaspoon salt
¼ teaspoon black pepper

Directions:

Preheat oven to 370F.

In a bowl combine the beef with egg, mustard seeds, ½ cup pureed tomatoes, apple cider vinegar, zucchini, onion, salt and pepper.

Grease 6-hole muffin tin with some coconut oil and divide the beef mixture between the holes.

Top each muffin meatloaf with remaining tomato puree and bake in preheated oven for 20 minutes. Allow to rest for 5 minutes before removing from the tin and serving.

Dinner

Thai Pork Salad

Serves: 4
Time: 15 minutes

Ingredients:

1 lb. ground pork
1 tablespoon extra-virgin olive oil
1 tablespoon chili paste
4 clove garlic, minced
2 spring onions, sliced
2 tablespoons lime juice, fresh
2 tablespoons chives
2 tablespoons fish sauce
¼ cup pine nuts
Some lettuce leaves

Directions:

Heat olive oil in large sauce pan; add the pine nuts and cook until toasted.

Add the ground pork and cook over medium heat until browned.

Add the fish sauce and chives and cook for 1 minute. Place the pork in a bowl, draining excess liquid.

Toss the pork with spring onions, garlic, chili paste and lime juice.

Spread few lettuce leaves on large plate and top with prepared pork.

Saffron Mussels

Serves: 2
Time: 15 minutes

Ingredients:

4 handfuls black mussels
8 oz. diced and seeded tomatoes
2 oz. fresh oregano, chopped
2 tablespoons coconut oil
2 oz. basil leaves, chopped
2 teaspoons minced garlic
Fresh ground salt and pepper
For the saffron sauce:
2 teaspoons saffron threads
4 cups fish stock
Fresh ground pepper
2 cups white wine

Directions:

Prepare the sauce; place the minced saffron in sauce pan; heat over low heat, until is heated through.

Add wine and fish stock; heat over medium heat and bring to simmer; simmer until sauce has reduced by 3/4.

Season with salt and pepper and set aside.

Prepare the mussels; heat the large skillet over medium-high heat and add the mussels with remaining ingredients and saffron sauce.

Toss the mussels with wooden spoon and cook until opened. Discard all unopened mussels before serving

Whole Roasted Lemon Chicken

Serves: 4
Time: 80 minutes

Ingredients:

2lb. whole chicken
3 lemons
3 garlic cloves, minced
¾ lb. carrots
2 tablespoons olive oil
2 tablespoons ginger powder
1 teaspoon salt
¾ teaspoon black pepper
3 sprigs rosemary, fresh

Directions:

Preheat oven to 400F.

Wash the chicken making sure that cavities are clean.

Place the chicken in baking dish and season with salt and pepper.

Zest the lemons and squeeze to get ¼ cup lemon juice. Combine the lemon juice with lemon zest. Add the garlic and garlic powder. Mix until combined.

Pour the mixture over chicken and top with rosemary sprigs.

Roast in the oven for 70 minutes or until juices run clear. Serve while still hot.

Chili Pork Stew

Serves: 4
Time: 70 minutes

Ingredients:

1.5 lb. pork shoulder meat, cut into 1 ½-inch pieces
2 tablespoons olive oil
1 onion, chopped
2.5oz. dried Mexican chilies, stemmed
1 tablespoon ancho chili powder
¼ tablespoon chili powder
1 teaspoon cumin, ground
½ teaspoon salt
½ teaspoon black pepper
½ tablespoon white vinegar
1 orange, juiced
4 cups water

Directions:

Heat the Mexican chilies in large pot; remove from the pot, place in a bowl and pour over water.

Drain chilies and reserve 2 cups of chili water. Place the chilies and water in food blender; add the ancho chili powder, chili powder, cumin and vinegar, salt, pepper and orange juice.

Puree the ingredients until smooth.

Heat olive oil in large sauce pot; season to taste with salt and pepper. Cook over medium-high heat until browned.

Add prepared chili sauce and cook for 45 minutes. Add the onions and cook for 10 minutes more. Serve while still hot.

Stuffed Snapper

Serves: 4
Time: 30 minutes

Ingredients:

4 red snappers, small
4 garlic cloves, sliced
2 lemons, sliced
2 sprigs dill
2 sprigs thyme
4 tablespoons olive oil

Salt and pepper – to taste

Directions:

Preheat oven to 450F.

Season the fish skin and the cavity with salt and pepper.

Stuff the fish with equal amounts of lemon slices, dill and thyme.

Transfer the fish onto greased baking dish and drizzle with olive oil. Bake the fish 20-25 minutes or until starts to flakes easily.

Beef and Peppers Stir-Fry

Serves: 4
Time: 20 minutes

Ingredients:

1 lb. beef flank steak, cut into stripes
3 tablespoons olive oil
1 tablespoon rice wine
1 green bell pepper, seeded, sliced into strips
2 tablespoons balsamic vinegar
1 onion, sliced
Salt and pepper – to taste
1 tablespoon sesame seeds

Directions:

Place the beef strips into bowl; add the rice wine and balsamic vinegar. Season with salt and pepper and toss to combine.

Heat 1 tablespoon olive oil in pan or wok. Add the coated beef and stir-fry for 2 minutes.

Remove the beef and place aside. Heat 1 tablespoon of oil in the same pan and add the onion; stir-fry for 2 minutes. Remove the onions and heat the remaining oil; add the pepper slices and stir-fry for 2 minutes.

Return beef and onions in the pan and add sesame seeds. Stir fry all for 1 minute and serve after.

Bacon Wrapped Avocado

Serves: 2
Time: 15 minutes

Ingredients:

2 pcs avocado, peeled, cut into 20 slices in total
20 pcs precooked bacon strips

Directions:

Preheat oven to 425F.

Wrap the bacon strips around the avocado slices and arrange onto baking sheet.

Bake the avocado for 10 minutes or until the bacon is crispy.

Serve while still hot with fresh salad.

Aromatic Moroccan Burgers

Serves: 4
Time: 20 minutes

Ingredients:

2lb. beef, ground, lean
2 teaspoons ground cumin
2 tablespoon cilantro, chopped
2 tablespoons parsley, chopped
½ teaspoon cumin
1 teaspoon chili powder
2 tablespoons olive oil

Directions:

Place the beef in a bowl. Add the cumin, cilantro, parsley, cumin and chili powder.

Mix all with clean hands.

Form 8 burgers from the mixture.

Heat olive oil in large skillet. Place half of the burgers in skillet and cook for 4 minutes per side. Repeat with remaining burgers.

Serve with fresh arugula salad.

Liver Meatballs

Serves: 4
Time: 20 minutes + inactive time

Ingredients:

0.5 lb. beef, ground, lean
0.5 lb. beef liver, ground
½ cup flax seeds meal
½ teaspoon smoked paprika
½ cup parsley, fresh, chopped
1 onion, chopped
1 teaspoon chili powder
3 garlic cloves, minced
Salt and pepper – to taste
1 tablespoon coconut oil, melted

Directions:

Combine the beef and liver with flax seeds meal, paprika, parsley, chili powder, garlic, salt and pepper in a bowl.

Heat the oil in skillet; add onion and cook for 8-10 minutes or until caramelized over medium-low heat. Place aside to cool and combine with beef mix. Cover and refrigerate for 1 hour.

Preheat oven to 400F and line baking sheet with parchment paper. Form the meatballs and arrange onto baking sheet.

Bake for 18-20 minutes or until cooked through. Serve with favorite sauce.

Dinner Pizza

Serves: 6
Time: 25 minutes

Ingredients:

2 cup cauliflower, cut into florets
4 eggs
2 tablespoons olive oil
1 tablespoon basil, dried
3 garlic cloves, minced
1 lb. Italian sausage, ground
½ cup tomato sauce, organic (or just puree 2 tomatoes)
2 tomatoes, sliced
3 scallions, sliced
Salt and pepper – to taste

Directions:

Place the cauliflower florets in food processor. Pulse to ground finely. Transfer in a bowl and add the eggs along with basil. Season with salt and pepper. Line the baking sheet with parchment paper and transfer the cauliflower mix onto baking sheet. Preheat oven to 370F and bake the cauliflower crust for 10 minutes.

Meanwhile, heat the large skillet over medium-high heat. Add the olive oil and once hot add the ground sausage with garlic and basil. Cook until sausage is browned.

Spread the tomato sauce over cauliflower crust and top with browned sausage. Top with tomatoes and scallions.

Bake the pizza and broil for 8 minutes. Slice and serve.

Crab Curry

Serves: 4
Time: 30 minutes

Ingredients:

2 whole crabs, 12 oz. meat in total
1 tablespoon coconut oil
1 teaspoon cinnamon
1 cup tomatoes, crushed
1 tablespoon coriander
1 teaspoon salt
2 bell pepper, red, chopped
1 tablespoon cumin
1 onion, chopped
1 teaspoon chili flakes
1/8 teaspoon cardamom, crushed
2 garlic cloves, minced

14 oz. coconut milk

Directions:

Rinse the crabs and pick out meat as much as possible.

Heat the coconut oil in sauce pot; add the cinnamon, cumin, chili flakes and cardamom. Cook for 3 seconds over medium-high heat. Add the onions and bell pepper and coat with the spice mixture.

Cook for 4-5 minutes, stirring and add the garlic. Add the fresh crab meat and tomatoes; stir well. Add the coconut milk and cook for 10 minutes. Serve warm.

Cauliflower Mash

Serves: 4
Time: 30 minutes

Ingredients:

1 cup coconut milk
1 tablespoon coconut oil
1 head cauliflower, cut into florets and roughly chopped
1 celery root, cut into cubes
2 garlic cloves, chopped
½ teaspoon salt
2 teaspoons basil, dried

Directions:

In a medium pot melt the coconut oil. Add garlic and cook for 1 minute. Add the coconut milk, cauliflower, celery, salt and basil.

Simmer for 25 minutes or until cauliflower is tender. Remove from the heat and puree using immersion blender.

Season additionally to taste and serve.

Stuffed Eggplants

Serves: 4
Time: 40 minutes

Ingredients:

2 pcs eggplant
¾ lb. beef, ground, lean
4 tablespoons coconut oil, melted
4 garlic cloves, minced
1 onion, chopped finely
1 teaspoon cinnamon
½ teaspoon salt
¼ teaspoon black pepper
200 oz. tomatoes, diced

Directions:

Preheat oven to 350F.

Cut the eggplant in half lengthwise; scoop out the seeds.

Melt 2 tablespoons coconut oil in skillet; place the eggplant, skin side down and cook for 5 minutes; flip over and cook for 5 minutes more.

Remove and place onto greased baking sheet. Heat 1 tablespoon of oil and add the onion; cook for 5 minutes. Add the garlic and cook for 1 minute more.

Add the beef and cook until browned. Add the diced eggplant flesh and cook for 5 minutes more.

Add the diced tomatoes and seasonings and cook for 5 minutes. Fill the eggplants with prepared mixture and drizzle with remaining oil. Bake in the oven for 25 minutes.

Serve while still hot, garnished with fresh parsley.

Wrapped Chicken Tights

Serves: 4
Time: 45 minutes

Ingredients:

8 slices bacon
4 chicken tights
1 teaspoon smoked paprika
½ teaspoon cumin

Directions:

Preheat oven to 375F.

Wash and pat-dry the chicken. Season the chicken with salt, cumin and smoked paprika. Wrap each chicken tight in 2 pieces of bacon slices.

Arrange onto baking sheet, lined with parchment paper. Bake for 40 minutes or until chicken is cooked through.

Serve after.

Lamb Meatballs

Serves: 12 meatballs
Time: 15 minutes

Ingredients:

1.5 lb. lamb, ground
2 garlic cloves, minced
½ teaspoon garlic powder
¾ teaspoon salt
¼ teaspoon black pepper
Zest of 1 lemon
4 slices lemon
2 tablespoons coconut oil, melted
2 teaspoons basil, dried

Directions:

Preheat oven to 400F.

In a bowl, combine the lamb meat, cloves, garlic powder, salt, black pepper, lemon zest and basil. Stir with clean hands and form meatballs from the prepared mixture.

Arrange the meatballs into oven-safe dish and top with lemon slices.

Drizzle with coconut oil and bake for 25 minutes or until cooked through.

Serve while still hot.

Tuna Cakes

Serves: 12 cakes
Time: 30 minutes

Ingredients:

10 oz. can tuna, packed in water, drained
2 eggs
1/3 cup scallions, chopped
2 tablespoons cilantro, minced
1 tablespoon jalapeno, seeded, minced
½ pcs lemon, zested
3 tablespoons coconut oil, melted
½ teaspoon red pepper flakes
1 ½ cups sweet potatoes, cooked, mashed
Salt and pepper – to taste

Directions:

Preheat oven to 350F and line 12-hole muffin tin with 1 tablespoon coconut oil.

In a bowl combine the tuna, eggs, scallions, cilantro, jalapeno, lemon zest, red pepper flakes and sweet potato mash.

Add the melted coconut oil, season to taste and stir until well combined. Transfer the mixture into greased muffin tin and smooth the surface using the back of spoon.

Bake the tuna cakes for 22-25 minutes. Place on wire rack to cool slightly before serving.

Chili Tilapia

Serves: 4
Time: 25 minutes

Ingredients:

1 lb. tilapia fillets
2 lb. asparagus, trimmed and cut into 1 ½-inch pieces
2 tablespoons chili powder
½ teaspoon garlic powder
3 tablespoons lemon juice
2 tablespoons olive oil
Salt and pepper – to taste

Directions:

Steam the asparagus in steaming basket placed over pot of simmering water (just 1-inch water) and steam for 4 minutes.

Combine the chili powder, garlic powder and at least two pinches of salt and pepper. Coat the fish with prepared mix and place aside.

Heat olive oil in large non-stick skillet; add the fish and cook for 6-7 minutes per side.

Remove the fish and serve on plate. Place the steamed asparagus in the same skillet and add lemon juice. Toss to combine and cook for 2 minutes.

Serve with fish.

Shrimps with Chile Paste

Serves: 4
Time: 15 minutes

Ingredients:

1 lb. shrimps, jumbo, deveined
2 tablespoons coconut oil, melted
1 teaspoon salt
1 teaspoon garlic powder
2 tablespoon almond flour
1 teaspoon black pepper
½ cup coconut cream
6 tablespoons chile paste
1 tablespoon apple cider vinegar

1 ½ tablespoons butter

Directions:

Devein and peel the shrimps; rinse under cold water and pat-dry with clean towel.

In a bowl combine the salt, pepper, almond flour and garlic powder. Add the shrimps and toss until shrimps are coated.

Heat the coconut oil in large skillet; add shrimps and cook for 2 minutes or until n longer pink.

In a small sauce pot combine the coconut cream, chile paste, cider vinegar and almond butter. Bring to gentle simmer and add in the shrimps. Remove from the heat and serve.

Spicy Salmon

Serves: 4
Time: 20 minutes

Ingredients:

1.25 lb. salmon fillets
½ lime, juiced and zested
2 tablespoons cilantro, chopped
1 ½ teaspoons sriracha sauce
½ teaspoon salt

Directions:

Preheat oven to 425F.

Combine the lime juice, cilantro and sriracha in a bowl.

Season the salmon fillets with salt and place into baking dish. Spread over the sriracha mix and roast the salmon for 15 minutes.

Serve while still hot.

Rich Shrimp-Avocado Salad

Serves: 4-6
Time: 10 minutes + inactive time

Ingredients:

2 lb. shrimps, deveined, peeled and broiled
2 avocados, peeled, stoned, diced
1 tablespoon red onion, sliced
¼ cup coconut oil, virgin, melted
1 teaspoon parsley
1 teaspoon mustard seeds, ground
½ teaspoon garlic powder
4 tablespoons lime juice
Salt and pepper – to taste

Directions:

In a large bowl combine the shrimps, avocados and red onion.

In separate, smaller bowl combine the coconut oil, parsley, mustard seeds, garlic powder, lime juice and salt and pepper to taste.

Drizzle the shrimps with prepared coconut oil mix and toss to combine.

Chill for 30 minutes before serving.

Dessert

Chocolate Mousse

Serves: 6
Time: 15 minutes

Ingredients:

4 avocados, ripe, peeled, stoned
4 bananas, unripe
½ cup cacao powder, unsweetened
1 cup coconut milk
2 tablespoons cacao nibs, raw
1 teaspoon vanilla extract

Directions:

In a food blender combine the avocados and bananas. Pulse until smooth.

Add the cacao powder, coconut milk and vanilla. Pulse until blended thoroughly.

Serve in bowls and top with cacao nibs.

Pumpkin Ice-Cream

Serves: 4
Time: 10 minutes + inactive time

Ingredients:

2 cups squash, cooked

14 oz. coconut milk
1 teaspoon almond extract
1 teaspoon cinnamon
1 pinch salt
2 tablespoons coconut oil, melted
2 egg yolks, pastured

Directions:

In a food blender combine all ingredients. Process until smooth.

Transfer the mixture into freezer-safe dish and place in the freezer for 2 hours. After 2 hours, stir using a fork and continue to freeze for 2 hours more.

Serve after.

Cacao Bites

Serves: 10 balls
Time: 10 minutes + inactive time

Ingredients:

1 cup almond butter
1 tablespoon cacao powder
½ cup shredded coconut, unsweetened
1 teaspoon vanilla paste

Directions:

Combine all ingredients in a bowl.

Stir mixture until all ingredients are blended thoroughly.

Form balls and place onto wide plate lined with parchment paper. Pop in the freezer for 15 minutes.

Serve after.

Vanilla-Lemon Cups

Serves: 12 cups
Time: 5 minutes + inactive time

Ingredients:

½ cup coconut oil, softened not melted
½ cup coconut butter
1 lemon, juiced and zested
1 teaspoon vanilla paste

Directions:

Line 12-hole muffin tin with paper cases.

In a bowl combine the coconut butter, coconut oil, lemon juice, lemon zest and vanilla paste until blended thoroughly.

Spoon the mixture into paper cups and pop in the freezer for 20 minutes.

Serve after.

5-minute Pumpkin Cake

Serves: 1
Time: 5 minutes

Ingredients:

1 egg
1 egg white
1 ½ tablespoons coconut flour
1 teaspoon vanilla
½ teaspoon cinnamon
¼ teaspoon baking soda
1pinch nutmeg
1 tablespoon pumpkin puree, organic
1 tablespoon coconut butter
1 tablespoon coconut milk
1 teaspoon almond butter
1 teaspoon cacao powder

Directions:

Prepare the chocolate topping; in a small bowl combine the coconut butter, coconut milk, almond butter, ½ teaspoon vanilla and cacao powder. Place aside.

In a large microwave-safe mug combine the egg, egg white, coconut flour ½ teaspoon vanilla, cinnamon, baking soda, nutmeg and pumpkin puree. Whisk all with a fork.

Place the mug in the microwave and microwave for 1 ½ - 2 ½ minutes on high.

While still hot, top with cacao mixture and serve.

Pumpkin Sweet Custard

Serves: 6
Time: 70 minutes

Ingredients:

1 cup pumpkin puree, organic
2 pinches nutmeg
1 teaspoon cinnamon
2 eggs
1 cup coconut milk
1 teaspoon vanilla paste

Directions:

Preheat oven to 350F.

Combine the pumpkin puree in a bowl with cinnamon and nutmeg.

In smaller bowl whisk the eggs with vanilla and coconut milk.

Combine these two mixtures and whisk until smooth. Spoon the mixture into six ramekins and place into baking dish. Fill the dish with water so it reaches the middle of ramekins.

Bake the custard for 60 minutes. Once baked remove from the oven and place aside to cool until it reaches room temperature. You can garnish with favorite fruits.

Thank You

I hope this book helped you to improve your eating habits, and you were able to achieve amazing results with the 21 Sugar Detox Diet.

After finishing the diet, you know, that you don't really need too much sugar, and you actually feel much better without it. The next step is, to stay in control of your sugar intake and not to fall back into sugar addiction.